Treadmill Desk Revolution:

The Easy Way to Lose Up To 50 Pounds in a Year – Without Dieting

by
Nick Loper
nickloper.com

Disclaimer

No part of this publication shall be reproduced, transmitted, or sold in whole or in part in any form, without the prior written consent of the author. All trademarks and registered trademarks appearing in this book are the property of their respective owners.

This book is intended for informational purposes only. The reader is responsible for his or her own actions.

The material in this book may include information, products, or services by third parties. All attempts have been made to verify the accuracy of this third party information, and neither the author nor the publisher assumes any responsibility for errors, omissions, or contrary interpretations of the material within.

Users of this guide are advised to do their own due diligence when it comes to making decisions and all information, products, and services that have been provided should be independently verified by your own qualified professionals. By reading this guide, you agree that the author is not responsible for the success or failure of your treadmill desk walking routine relating to any information presented in this book.

Treadmill Desk Revolution: The Easy Way to Lose Up To 50 Pounds in a Year – Without Dieting

Introduction

Our bodies weren't built to sit, yet that is how we spend the majority of our waking hours. Our increasingly sedentary lifestyles have led to a host of health issues, including heart disease, obesity, and premature death.

But it doesn't have to be that way.

Right now in our midst is a group of pioneering individuals and companies who have made a conscious shift in the way they work. While the rest of the world is getting sicker, these innovators are melting inches off their waistlines, losing weight, and creating healthier lives.

What's their secret?

It's simple: **walking**.

They have refashioned their workstations with treadmills and walk while they work.

Sounds a little crazy, right?

Well, every good idea seems a little crazy at first. We are just now on the forefront of the treadmill desk revolution, and this book aims to:

- Paint a picture of the long-term dangers of sitting, in contrast to standing and walking.

- Review some of the dramatic success stories from current treadmill desk "jockeys."

- Show how you and your company can join in.

Nomadic Roots

Throughout evolution, our ancestors were on the move. They had no comfy couches and apartments; they had to keep moving to find food, water, and shelter – and to avoid predators.

Today we're our own most dangerous predator. The perils of the modern life are far more likely to kill us than an unforeseen lion attack.

Early humans walked 6-10 miles a day – the equivalent of crossing North America over the course of a year! In contrast, the average American today walks just 3 miles, with many of us not even reaching that distance.

Given our ancestry and unique two-legged construction, it seems clear our bodies were built to be upright and in motion. And despite how amazingly adaptable we are as a species, there is mounting evidence that the farther we stray from nature's intended use, the higher our risk for developing an array of physiological ailments.

Settling Down

For millennia, the trend has been toward less walking.

We started farming, domesticating animals, and building permanent settlements.

But for most people, work was still *work*. Survival and employment meant **physical labor** for all but a few members of society.

In fact, as late as the 1860s more than half the American population still lived and worked on farms. Compare that to less than 3% today.

Removing the physical *work* from work is not a new idea – we've always sought out new inventions and efficiencies to make our lives easier – but the trend accelerated with the Industrial Revolution and kicked into hyperspeed with the Computer Revolution.

Our generation spends more time sitting than any one before us – as much as 9 hours a day or more! We are a product of our environment; we have longer commutes, spend more time at our desks, and log more TV hours than ever before.

These habits are reinforced from an early age. Just think about how many times as a child you were told to "sit still!"

This lifestyle change means we're burning far fewer calories than our parents and grandparents did. Over the course of a week, we may burn 1000 calories less than the average person 50 years ago. Add that to diet filled with sugary, starchy, and processed foods (volumes have been written dissecting the evils of our modern diet; it's far beyond the scope of this book), and it's a recipe for disaster.

What To Do About It?

Even the fanciest Hermann Miller chair can't protect our bodies from undoing thousands of years of evolutionary biology. And we can't exactly go back to being hunters and gatherers either.

So what's the answer?

Since we can't change the work that needs to get done, we need to change how we interface with that work.

That's where the treadmill desk comes in.

Ready to join the revolution?

Table of Contents

Success Story #1: The Pants of Wrath

The tipping point for Virginia-based software developer Brian Slick came when he had to purchase a pair of pants in a size he **swore he would never buy**. Around the same time in early 2012, a colleague had made a treadmill desk of his own and was reporting "pretty significant weight loss," Brian says.

Brian readily admits, "I'm not really good about regular exercise or going to the gym. I needed some way to get exercise while doing work." The treadmill desk was a natural solution.

The Desk

One challenge was finding a treadmill desk model at an acceptable price point. Brian discovered the LifeSpan TR1200-DT online for around $1299 (now closer to $1500), which included free shipping.

He customized the desk with an add-on shelf in the back to elevate the monitor to eye level.

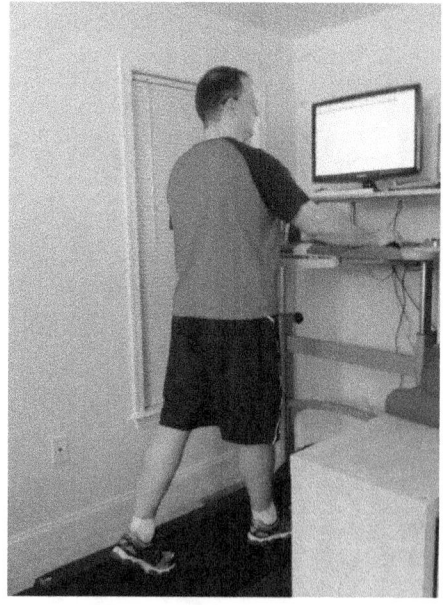

Brian at his LifeSpan treadmill desk

The Results

In just over a year of walking, Brian has lost **50 pounds**.

And those pants he swore he'd never buy? They're now "significantly too large," Brian says with a smile.

The treadmill desk appears to be creating change in other areas of health as well. "Since getting the treadmill, I've only been sick once, and that happened while traveling over the holidays," Brian explains. "I can also go outside and walk around much quicker than I could before I got the treadmill."

The Miles

In a typical week, Brian racks up almost 40 miles at the treadmill desk.

However, not every mile has been pain-free. "I probably ramped up too quickly," Brian says while discussing the pain he suffered in his feet. Of course, "the net result has still been worth it," he adds, but suggests new treadmill desk walkers start slow or consult a doctor before starting.

The Speed

1.2 mph

The Shoes

"I'm partial to Asics," Brian explains, showing off his sneakers. The model he wears is called GEL-Nimbus.

About Brian Slick

Brian Slick is the founder of BriTer Ideas LLC, a contract iPhone and iPad application development firm in Northern Virginia. You can follow along with his treadmill desk adventure and weight loss progress at his blog: clingingtoideas.blogspot.com.

Sitting by the Numbers

Today, fewer than 20% of our jobs require any kind of physical exertion. What's been labeled as the service economy could also be called the **sitting economy**. We work with our brains and our fingers instead of with our arms, legs, and backs.

Office workers spend the majority of their time sitting behind a desk or commuting.

More than half the population sits 9 hours or more every day. And while sitting is more prevalent in developed economies, it truly is a planet-wide phenomenon.

Outside of the workplace, sitting is our most popular pastime. A long-term Australian health study found the average adult spends fully 90% of their leisure time sitting down. That's why they call it leisure time, right?

Consider how many hours a day you spend in a car, in a chair, or on the couch.

If you sleep 8 hours a night, that leaves 16 hours left in the day. Of that time, we spent most of it on our butts. In 2010, a UK study found Britons sitting on average more than 14 and a half hours every day!

We're not much better; Americans sit an average of nearly 11 hours a day according to recent study.

It's easy for the hours to add up, even during innocent, normal activities. While this book will focus on reducing sitting during work hours by using a treadmill desk, think of where other opportunities may lie to reduce your sitting time:

- Eating meals

- Commuting to and from work

- Watching TV

- Surfing the Internet

The Bureau of Labor Statistics found the average American watching 2.8 hours of TV every day, or nearly 20 hours a week. (A 2012 Nielsen report puts the number closer to 34 hours a week – **almost another full-time job!**) You can imagine how a small change in habit could make a big impact on total sedentary hours.

But these numbers don't mean much without understanding the dire consequences of the siting lifestyle. In the following section, we'll explore some of the frightening dangers of extended sitting.

Success Story #2: The Biggest Losers

When Barry Lipsett first saw a treadmill desk while visiting a customer's office in late 2012, he knew his company should have them too. As president of Charles River Apparel, he orchestrated the installation of 3 treadmill desks at their Boston-area headquarters in January 2013.

The Desks

Charles River Apparel installed 3 LifeSpan TR1200 treadmill desks and placed them in different locations around the office. The machines cost around $1400 apiece, and also required a small additional infrastructure investment of extra computer hardware and phone equipment to reside permanently at the treadmill workstations.

At first, employees were a bit hesitant to begin using these new contraptions. But rather than have his investment collect dust, Lipsett **led by example** and began using them himself, even holding meetings around the treadmill desk while he walked.

Before long, other workers jumped on and it soon became socially acceptable to use the treadmill desks, which are available on a first-come-first-served basis to all Charles River Apparel employees. Now, all three workstations are routinely in use all day long.

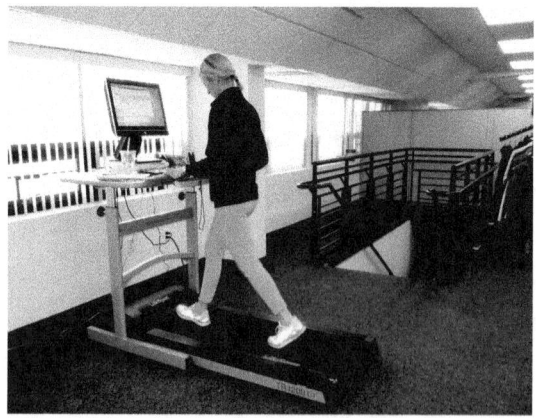

A Charles River Apparel employee walking the day away

The Results

Employees are participating in a "Biggest Loser"-style competition to see who can drop the most weight this year, with significant prize money on the line. To sweeten the deal, Charles River has offered to match the employee contributions, doubling the pot for the winner.

The treadmill desks are an integral part of the weight loss strategy and goals for the participants. Vice President of Marketing, Vanessa Keefe, is down 10 pounds in just over 3 months, but she explains she's not even the frontrunner.

"One co-worker is down **nearly 40 pounds** already!" she says, by walking during the day and also hitting the gym after work.

The presence of the treadmill desks combined with the proactive leadership from the company's management has helped foster a renewed focus on health in the office.

The Miles

Together, Charles River employees have trekked more than 2100 miles so far this year -- all from the comfort of their office. That's enough to get them from their Boston-area headquarters all the way to Salt Lake City, Utah!

The Shoes

Keefe explains the office dress code is pretty casual, and that sneakers are acceptable to wear to work. Those who choose to wear dressier shoes often bring a pair of walking shoes so they can get in their treadmill time as well.

About Charles River Apparel

Charles River Apparel is a family-owned and operated company that manufactures superior quality clothing and outerwear for the whole family. They've been recognized by Boston Magazine as a "Best Place to

Work," and named one of the Top 10 Small Businesses in the state of Massachusetts. The 60-person company generates annual revenue in excess of $30 million.

Is Sitting Killing Us?

But it's so comfortable!

Unfortunately, a growing body of scientific evidence suggests our sedentary lifestyle is contributing to host of modern ailments including heart disease, obesity, diabetes, and cancer.

Put another way, the more you sit, the sooner you'll die.

Researchers in Australia reached that alarming conclusion after studying the habits of more than 200,000 people. In the end, they found a direct correlation between sitting hours and shorter life expectancies.

But this research is hardly cutting edge. Italian physician Bernardino Ramazzini made strikingly similar observations 300 years ago:

> *"Those who sit at their work ... suffer from their own particular diseases. These workers ... suffer from general ill-health and an excessive accumulation of unwholesome humors caused by their sedentary life."* – Diseases of Workers, 1713

He advised patients to get some exercise to "counteract the harm done by many days of sedentary life." See how far medicine has advanced?

More Deadly Than Cigarettes?

A high-profile study found those who sat 6 hours per day – not an unreasonable "average" – effectively had a lifespan nearly 5 years shorter than non-sitters.

But everyone sits some of the time. This book is about becoming more aware of our idle hours and making the necessary changes that could literally save our lives.

Researchers framed the issue another way, saying that each hour of "TV time" as adults could end up costing us 21 minutes in life expectancy. For the sake of comparison, smoking a cigarette was found to cost just 11 minutes.

Heart Disease

Starting in the mid-20th Century, we began to link sitting and overall heart health. A British study found higher instances of cardiovascular disease in sedentary workers, like bus drivers, than those with jobs that required them to stand, like postal workers.

A more recent study split participants into two groups: those who logged more than 4 hours of idle sitting time (watching TV, sitting at the computer), and those who logged less than 2. Even after controlling for other factors like smoking and high blood pressure, the group with more sitting time experienced a 125% greater risk for heart disease and heart attacks.

Men in the sedentary group had a 64% greater risk of dying from heart disease than those in the active group.

An occupational study found workers who mostly stood at work had half the rate of cardiovascular disease than those who mostly sat. After two hours of sitting, participants noted a 20% decrease in good cholesterol.

The World Health Organization attributes "physical inactivity" to 30% of heart disease cases.

It seems our heart is trying to tell us something: **get up and move**.

Obesity

Beyond diet, your daily activity is a strong predictor of your body mass index, or BMI. In the past 30 years, reported "sitting time" in the US has increased a modest 8% but obesity rates have nearly tripled.

Obviously there are a number of factors that go into maintaining a healthy weight, but clearly our increasingly sedentary lives are not helping the issue. To support this, one study found that overweight individuals sat an average of 2.5 hours more each day than their thinner peers.

Almost as soon as we sit down, our **metabolism slows to a crawl –** burning just one calorie per minute.

During long idle periods, our bodies dramatically slow down key enzymes that help break down fat. That may be good news for animals in hibernation, but it's bad news for us.

Diabetes

Along with the dire health risks above comes an increased danger of diabetes. Long periods of inactivity reduce insulin effectiveness by 24%.

"When we sit down there is an absence of muscle contractions," explains Professor David Dunstan, of the Baker IDI Heart and Diabetes Institute. "These contractions are required for the body to clear blood glucose and blood fats from the blood stream."

Inactivity is the "main cause" of 27% of diabetes cases, according to the World Health Organization.

Cancer

In 2011, The American Institute for Cancer Research conducted a large meta study of over 200 cancer papers. The study linked physical inactivity to more than 43,000 cases of colon cancer and almost 50,000 cases of breast cancer, and reached the conclusion that excessive idle time greatly increased one's risk for developing cancer.

Physiological Risks

Beyond the life-threatening maladies above (as if those weren't bad enough!), sitting also carries a number of risks to your musculoskeletal system.

For example, a normal seated position has your feet on the floor under your body, which contracts the hamstring muscles on the backs of your legs. Maintaining this position over time can shorten the muscles, leading to tightness and inflexibility, and making you more prone to injury. Hamstring problems have also been linked to lower back pain.

Similarly, the hip flexors on the front of your legs can become contracted and shortened by long periods of sitting.

In addition, excessive sitting with poor posture – hunched over a computer, for example – can lead to back, neck, and shoulder problems.

But I Exercise!

One of the scariest bits of data in these frightening studies is that the recommended 30 minutes of daily exercise does NOT seem to counteract the negative effects of sitting the rest of the time. Even if you exercise, the research suggests a heavy-sitting lifestyle makes you 40% more likely to die within 15 years.

To be fair, exercise is still important for heart and muscle health, as well as mental clarity – but is not a miracle cure for the diseases of sitting.

Success Story #3: The Disappearing Act

Francine Dittrich is a vocational case manager for an insurance company in Portland, Oregon. When her company installed 3 treadmill desks in their offices, she knew it was the perfect opportunity to try and lose weight.

"I had a strong desire to change my lifestyle," she explains. With the treadmill desk readily available and the support of her co-workers, Francine began walking in the spring of 2011.

The Desk

Francine's employer, Standard Insurance Company, installed several Steelcase Walkstation treadmill desks throughout their offices for workers to reserve and use. The one Francine used is located in a facility known as the Workplace Possibilities Center, which showcases equipment that helps people stay at work who might otherwise be unable to due to pain or discomfort caused by their working environment.

The Steelcase brand among the more well-known treadmill desk manufacturers, with several models starting around $2000.

The Results

"I lost **60 pounds** while using the Walkstation and watching the quantity of food I consumed." After that, Francine continued her amazing transformation by incorporating other activities into her lifestyle while continuing to walk at work, and dropped another 55 pounds.

"**The Walkstation helped change my life**," Francine glows.

In less than 2 years, Dittrich cut her weight **almost in half**, going from 254 pounds to 138. She's down from a size 26 to a size 10 petite.

The Miles

Perhaps even more amazing is the relatively limited time spent on the treadmill. "I don't usually keep track using miles; I use time," Francine explains. "I usually walk an hour a day, depending on my workload."

The Speed

"When starting out, I walked at just over 1 mph and kept increasing it week after week." Now a seasoned treadmill desk veteran, Francine walks at 2 mph, which is the top speed setting on the Walkstation.

The Shoes

Aside from being overweight, Francine struggled with painful plantar fasciitis. She swears by her Brooks sneakers, which is the brand she's worn from the beginning.

About Francine Dittrich

Francine Dittrich is a Vocational Case Manager at Standard Insurance Company. The Standard is proud to be on the cutting edge of health initiatives in the workplace such as their Workplace Possibilities program. Francine's inspiring story was picked up by the Associated Press in 2013.

Enter the Treadmill Desk

A California Pioneer

In 1996, Seth Roberts created the first known treadmill desk. The UC Berkeley professor of psychology began his experiment by simply raising his office desk so he could stand while working. Where did the idea come from? "I ... believe that sitting is bad for you," said Roberts.

Almost immediately he found an unexpected benefit: he was sleeping more soundly at night. For years he'd struggled with restless nights and waking up too early in the morning.

And since standing was better than sitting, walking would probably be even better than standing. "After I discovered how much standing a lot helped my sleep, then I got a treadmill," Roberts said.

And the treadmill desk revolution was born.

It should be noted that Roberts was not out to lose weight, but rather wanted to create a more "stone age" environment in the modern office. He reasoned that our ancestors used their standing and walking muscles far more than we do today, so it would be a worthwhile experiment to see what would happen if we emulated them, instead of forcing our bodies into sedentary roles they largely weren't built for.

A New Champion

Despite Roberts' innovative and pioneering efforts, he was not the champion the cause needed in order to gain widespread awareness. In fact, he primarily used the desk for standing and stopped using the treadmill portion of the desk entirely after a couple years of his colleagues complaining about the noise.

Dr. James Levine, an endocrinologist at the Mayo Clinic is widely credited with bringing the treadmill desk into the mainstream.

In 2005, Dr. Levine fashioned a makeshift contraption by attaching a bedside hospital tray to a $400 treadmill. His invention sprung from his work on ways to improve metabolism and weight loss.

A leading researcher in non-exercise activity thermogenesis (NEAT), Levine was looking for out-of-the-box ways to address the "standing gap" – the discovery that thin people spent an average of an extra 2 and half hours on their feet each day than their overweight counterparts.

Since the workplace is where many of us do a lot of sitting, it was a natural progression to rethink the way we work.

Perhaps because of the novelty of the invention or perhaps because of the increased attention on obesity, the treadmill desk idea was covered in several media outlets including CNN, Good Morning America, and USA Today.

Before long, individuals all over the country were building their own treadmill desks, and companies rushed to create new mobile workstations to address the needs of this exciting new market. Early adopters were vocal about their new way of working while walking, and the movement began to take hold.

After all, an invention that could be likened to a human hamster wheel is nothing if not a conversation starter, right?

Success Story #4: The $100 Treadmill Desk

Alfred Poor is a technology expert, author and public speaker based in Philadelphia. He started using a treadmill desk in 2011.

"I was turning 60 that year," he explains, "and I was getting more aches and pains." As a result of the down economy, Poor was forced to spend more time at work and his exercise routine no longer fit into his schedule.

He found himself falling asleep in his chair and losing productivity.

"I discovered the concept of a walking desk on the web, and I knew I had to make one for myself."

The Desk

Lacking budget for expensive new office furniture, Alfred went the do-it-yourself route, and ended up putting the whole thing together for less than $100.

"My first step was to scavenge a discarded hollow-core closet door. Then I bought a used treadmill on Craigslist. It took me about a week to find one conveniently close and under my target price."

He cut the door down to six feet and used some inexpensive lumber to make the framework. Next, he securely mounted the desk surface to the treadmill itself for stability.

"I also removed the control panel," Alfred explained. This allowed him to elevate the panel so it would sit flush with the desk surface and make the desk portion easier to detach if it ever needs to be moved.

In the end, the total costs were $75 for the treadmill, $10 for wood, and $5 for some cable connectors used to extend the control panel.

The Results

So far, Alfred has lost **11 pounds**. This has reduced his waist size by several inches. And beyond the weight loss and outward appearance, he says, "The biggest gains are in **core strength and muscle tone**."

"And I have more stamina," he adds. "I believe I'm more alert and think better when I'm walking."

The Miles

An average of 6-8 miles a day, or 30-40 miles a week.

The Speed

"I started off walking almost all day at 1 mph and a 5 degree incline. Now I'm at 1.2 mph and a 6 degree incline." The incline adds to the challenge and gives your leg muscles a better workout.

About Alfred Poor

Alfred Poor's writing has been seen in PC Magazine, PC World, and dozens of other print and online outlets. As a leading expert in the area of information display, he has reached an audience of millions through his writing and public speaking. He is also the author of *7 Success Secrets that Every College Student Needs to Know*.

Benefits of Walking While Working

Walking while working carries a number of benefits, both to your short- and long-term health, and to your work itself. The biggest advantage is simply **extending your life**. Walking at work – or simply standing – greatly reduces your risk of developing the "sitting diseases" discussed earlier.

Walking 10,000 steps a day can result in 90% reduction in heart attacks and a nearly 70% reduction in the rate of stroke, according to the American Heart Association. The American Cancer Society reports 30-70% lower cancer rates, and the American Diabetes Association data cites a 50% reduction in Type 2 diabetes.

Aside from outliving their idle colleagues, treadmill desk users enjoy lower cholesterol, reduced blood pressure, improved circulation, and faster metabolisms.

Lose Weight

The one reason that draws many people to try a treadmill desk is the promise of losing weight. And in fact, it can be a tremendously effective way to shed those extra pounds without dieting and without going to the gym.

Dr. Levine estimates the average person could burn an extra 100-150 calories an hour, depending on their weight and the speed they set the treadmill to. Most treadmills have a calorie display on their control panel, and it can become quite addicting to watch the calories burn off over the course of the day.

Without any change to diet, treadmill desk walkers who are burning an incremental 500-1000 calories a day could stand to **lose 25-50 pounds in a year**. As we've seen in some of the examples in this book, the results are dramatic and life-changing, and are being achieved by regular people who decided to make just one small change in the way they work.

Reduce Stress

Physical activity like walking triggers the release of endorphins in the brain, which improve our moods and reduce stress. One study found that taking a walk had a calming effect similar to a mild tranquilizer.

In side-by-side comparisons, treadmill desk walkers had higher self-esteem and fewer instances of depression than their non-walking peers.

Cardiologist Dr. James Rippe has studied the health benefits of walking and found even low-intensity walking had a profound positive impact on one's anxiety levels and overall feelings of stress.

In the workplace, that can result in happier and more productive employees.

Improve Productivity

Surprisingly, walking can make it easier to concentrate. Just how runners and other athletes talk about being "in the zone" – often described as a state of "flow" in positive psychology – treadmill desk walkers offer up a similar experience.

"I thought it was ridiculous until I tried it," said 49 year old Terri Krivosha, a partner at a Minnesota law firm. She went on to explain how walking helped filter out distractions and keep her focused throughout the day. "Walking takes care of the A.D.D. part," she added with a smile.

This example was replicated on a larger scale by a 2011 Lancaster University study that tracked the walking habits of more than 700 US and UK employees in a variety of fields. Those who took 10,000 steps in a day (tracked by a pedometer) reported significantly higher levels of workplace productivity. The same workers also noted improved job satisfaction, self-confidence, and concentration.

10,000 steps is the rough equivalent of 1.5 – 2 hours of treadmill desk walking time. **It doesn't take much!**

It should be noted that even the simple act of removing chairs from conference rooms can have a similar productivity-boosting effect. Several years ago, a Los Angeles company ditched the chairs and found their meetings were over in half the time. Attendees tended to stay on topic more and make their points with a greater sense of urgency than when they were comfortably sitting.

A Sense of Accomplishment

Beyond the physical benefits, an important benefit not always cited in studies is the sense of pride and accomplishment experienced by treadmill desk walkers.

It's like, "I did great work today, AND I walked 6 miles!" That's why you see so many people tracking their steps and their miles. The distance is a well-earned badge of honor above and beyond the normal workday.

Success Story #5: The Walking Office

In 2007, Dr. Levine and the Mayo Clinic set out to test their theories about physical movement in the workplace on a larger scale. They found a perfect partner in nearby Minneapolis, Minnesota with Salo, a financial staffing and consulting agency.

Salo agreed to install several treadmill desks in their office and measure the impact on employee health.

The Desks

Salo installed a bank of 6 Steelcase Details Walkstations in an open area for workers to use. Employees can reserve time in advance in 2-hour increments or use the machines as they become available.

Among the all-in-one treadmill desk solutions, the Walkstation is a very popular model and costs around $4000. Because it is specifically designed for office environments, it is built to withstand hours of use each day and run quietly to minimize noise pollution.

As Salo has grown, they've added more treadmill desks, and now have 11 in total. The company even added 4 treadmill desks to their conference room, which face each other to facilitate walking meetings.

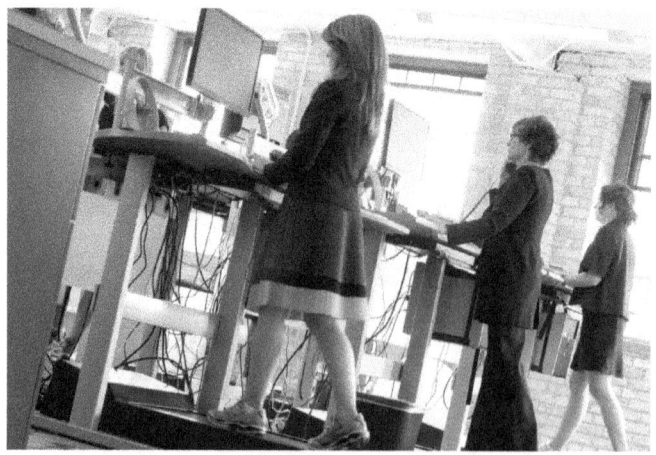

Salo employees laying down the miles

The Results

For six months, 18 Salo employees rotated on and off the new treadmill desks, walking an average of 3 hours a day. Cholesterol was down across the board and harmful triglycerides dropped an average of 37% for the participants.

Among the new treadmill desk walkers was Director of Operations and Administration, Craig Dexheimer, who lost **25 pounds** during the six-month study.

Not bad, "For just going to work!" he says.

On top of that, employees were more productive; the company produced record revenues during the study! Dexheimer credits a more dynamic and energized workplace.

The Miles

For Craig, the usage varies day-to-day depending on the work that has to get done. Still, he makes a point to try and jump on as often as he can and at least get a couple miles in.

He sets the speed to 2 mph, which is the maximum setting for the Walkstation.

The Shoes

Even though Salo maintains a professional office environment, employees are encouraged to walk during the work-day. Some saunter in their dress shoes but others bring in tennis shoes for comfort.

"I've got a pair of black Nikes," Dexheimer explains. "They actually don't look too bad with a suit."

About Salo

From their Minneapolis and Chicago offices, Salo provides financial and accounting staffing services for project-based work, interim assignments, and permanent placement. The company was founded in 2002 and has been on the forefront of the employee health and treadmill desk movements.

How it Works

Walking while working can take some getting used to. In this section, we'll cover the physical and technical considerations, as well as some best practices for treadmill desk walkers.

The Set Up

For proper desk height, make sure the monitor is at eye level, and the keyboard and mouse can be used comfortably. It may be a matter of personal preference, but your wrists can comfortably rest and type at roughly the level of your hips. This way you can maintain a healthy upright posture and keep from hunching down to see the screen.

For best results, you'll need to use an external monitor apart from your laptop or keyboard. Using only the laptop by itself might make either the screen too low or force your hands to be too high.

The other thing to consider is slowing down the mouse speed, especially at the beginning. Because your arms and hands will be moving a bit more than you're used to, a reduced mouse speed can help improve click accuracy.

Start Slow

Beginning treadmill desk walkers should start at just 1 mph. It will seem painfully slow, but this leisurely pace will get you used to walking while working and re-engage your potentially atrophied foot, calf, and ankle muscles.

Aside from speed, you might want to limit your treadmill time initially. Even though it's just walking, it will be a shock to your body if you try to go from 0 miles a day to 10 right out of the gate.

It takes some practice to be able to type and click effectively, all while walking in a straight line. Start slow and ramp up as you feel comfortable.

Normally, you'll want to keep it at a pace where you don't break a sweat and don't get out of breath, although for certain tasks that don't require your direct input (reading or watching a video, for example), feel free to crank up the speed and burn some extra calories.

Take Breaks

If you feel tired or are having a hard time focusing, it's totally OK to take a break. In fact, one beautiful thing about a treadmill desk is once the belt stops it simply becomes a standing desk.

Also, you won't want to throw out your old desk right away either. Having a traditional sit-down desk as a backup is a great strategy and makes you appreciate the comfort of sitting that much more.

Then, when you're ready to start walking again, just turn the treadmill back on and jump to it!

Footwear

Comfortable walking shoes are absolutely required. For certain office environments, that might mean packing one pair of "dressy" shoes and one pair of athletic shoes. If your feet aren't prepared for walking several hours each day, they will let you know in a hurry with painful hot spots, soreness, and blisters.

Socks

Socks can sometimes be an afterthought but they are very important in preventing hot spots and blisters. Regular cotton socks can trap heat and moisture, and lose their softness over time.

Instead, consider wearing running socks that are specifically made for athletic performance. They will typically be made from polyester and nylon, which is more form-fitting and moisture-wicking for extended walking.

Success Story #6: The Doctor is In (Motion)

Dr. Lauren Streicher is an author and gynecologist based in Chicago. She began her treadmill desk adventure in 2012 after attending a medical conference on health and obesity. Among other material covered, a presenter outlined the deadly risks of sitting and how people could fight back by using a standing desk or a treadmill desk.

The Desk

When she got home from the conference, she ordered a TrekDesk from Amazon for around $400. It is a large and sturdy piece of furniture designed to fit over a treadmill, which Dr. Streicher already had in her home.

After falling in love with walking while working, she recently upgraded to a beautiful new TreadDesk model for around $2000. The new desk is more compact so it fits in a more desirable room in her house, and has an electronically adjustable height mechanism.

The Results

Before the treadmill desk, Dr. Streicher experienced neck pains and stiffness after a long day in front of the computer. "I just felt crummy," she said about sitting all day.

Once she started walking though, the neck pain went away and she also noticed her body and muscles felt more toned. To get the ergonomics right, Dr. Streicher installed an external keyboard so she could keep the laptop screen elevated and her head up.

The Miles

An average of 20-30 miles a week, but as many as 8 or 9 miles in day when she's really in a groove.

The Speed

The treadmill desk speed varies based on the work she's doing. "If I am writing, I keep it at 1.5 mph," she explains. "Editing, 2.0 mph. Conference calls, doing interviews, etc. 3.0 mph."

About Dr. Lauren Streicher

Dr. Streicher is an Assistant Clinical Professor of Obstetrics and Gynecology at Northwestern University.

As a leading expert on women's health, she has appeared on a number of TV outlets including Oprah, The Today Show, and The Dr. Oz Show. She is the author of *The Essential Guide to Hysterectomy*, and has new book on sexual health due out in 2014.

Treadmill Desk Negatives

Although we've explored many of the benefits of treadmill desk walking, this book would not be complete if it didn't address the negative side as well.

Noise

Treadmill desks are unquestionably noisier than traditional desks. Even operating at low speeds, the belt, motor, and footsteps all combine to create a bit of noise pollution in the workplace. For home-based workers, it's usually not the end of the world, but in an office environment it can be a distraction for others – even though it could be considered fairly consistent white noise.

Since most treadmills were built for gyms or for home workouts, the noise they create was something of an afterthought for the manufacturers. Now, with more and more models being repurposed or intentionally built for offices, quietness is becoming a more important feature.

Later, we'll take a look at some treadmill models that are among the quietest on the market.

Space

The physical footprint of the treadmill desk may be larger than the traditional desk it replaces. If your office is going to add a bank of treadmill desks in addition to the regular sitting desks, there are obviously some space calculations that need to be made.

A popular set-up is for the company to install several treadmill desks in a common area so employees can jump on or off as they want. An alternative is to place them in different locations throughout the office (as space allows) so that every department can have equal access.

Weight

Treadmills are extremely heavy and awkward to move. Thankfully, many are foldable and have wheels, but can still be difficult to maneuver up stairs and around corners, especially in a home office set-up.

Insurance

One concern among employers is the risk of increased insurance rates if they install treadmill desks. While the company may end up saving on health insurance premiums as the result of a healthier workforce, their workplace insurance costs may increase if the insurer views the treadmills as a potential source of injury in the office.

Note: No documented cases of insurance rates increasing were found at press time.

Cost

Treadmill desks can range in price from less than $200 on the cheap do-it-yourself end, all the way up to $4000 for premium specialty high-end models.

Even though the long-term health benefits greatly outweigh the investment, there is an initial cost that may be a barrier for some companies.

Not a Good Fit for Every Job

Some jobs and tasks are better suited to walking than others. For example, reading and responding to emails, doing spreadsheet work, writing, and making phone calls can all be easily accomplished while walking at a treadmill desk.

However, other tasks that require precision mouse-work, like graphic design, will be considerably more difficult. Indeed, the University of Tennessee found up to an 11% deterioration in fine-motor skills, such as mouse clicking, among treadmill desk walkers.

Similarly, physically writing pen-on-paper style can be a challenge. It can be done, but takes some practice to write legibly to the same caliber as your non-walking self.

Productivity Loss?

Not everyone works as productively while they're walking. For certain users, Dr. Levine's Mayo Clinic found that typing speed and accuracy was reduced by 16% compared with typing at a standard desk.

Not a Substitute for Exercise

To be sure, walking even a couple hours on a treadmill desk is better than sitting idle all day at a traditional desk. However, that walking is not a substitute for real exercise.

It's still important for your cardiovascular health and your muscle strength to go out and break a sweat.

Success Story #7: The Energy Crisis Solved

Susan Baroncini-Moe is a business and marketing strategy consultant based in Indianapolis, Indiana. After reading a series of articles on the dangers of sedentary work, she decided it was time to take action.

She began her treadmill desk journey in the spring of 2012.

The Desk

Susan and her husband, Leo, designed and built the treadmill desk themselves. The treadmill itself is a Horizon T101, which runs between $600-700 brand new.

The desk portion is a tall wooden desk that spans over the treadmill cross bars. The cost for the necessary materials was less than $50.

To still be able to access the controls, they actually removed the control panel and mounted it directly to the desk. Susan and Leo added supports to stabilize the base. "Since we didn't touch the electronics themselves, I'm pretty sure the warranty is still valid," Susan explains.

The treadmill desk immediately became part of the family. It's even been given a name: Wendy. "Wendy has her own speakers, built-in fan, and cup holders," Susan adds. "Basically, she's tricked out."

The Results

"When I'm consistently working on the treadmill desk, my weight does drop, but most importantly, I keep **sustained energy** throughout the day." She notes, "I don't have that 2:00 PM slump I used to have."

The treadmill can give a boost of energy when working with clients and in general lead to improved productivity.

Susan also mentions that her stress level seems to drop while walking, which was an unexpected benefit.

The Miles

"In a typical week, I walk around 20-30 miles, depending on what I'm doing."

The Speed

Susan says her average speed is probably around 1.5 mph, noting that she worked her way up to that rate. She adds, "I can still type at 2.5 mph, but that gets a little dangerous!"

The Shoes

"I'm still trying to decide about the best pair of walking shoes. I've tried Brooks, Nike Free, and (embarrassingly) Crocs."

About Susan Baroncini-Moe

Susan Baroncini-Moe is an author, business strategist, podcaster, and Guinness World Record holder. (She holds the record for longest uninterrupted live webcast!) As a speaker, she has shared the stage with Michael Gerber, Bob Burg, Chris Brogan, and many more. Her book *Business in Blue Jeans* is due out in June 2013.

Build or Buy?

To build a treadmill desk or to buy one? For many prospective work-walkers, that is the question. In this section we'll explore the pros and cons of each option.

Buying

Obviously, if you have the cash, it will be quicker and easier to just order up a ready-made treadmill desk. However, as the demand for these contraptions grows, there are more and more choices on the market. Some are quite basic while others have all the bells and whistles imaginable – with the price tag to match.

Later we'll take a look at some of the popular treadmill desk models and help you find the one that is the best fit for you.

Building

Building your own treadmill desk is a fantastic option and can be done for a very low budget. Going the do-it-yourself route is very popular among home-office walkers and is well-suited to the experimental roots of the treadmill desk movement.

When Professor Roberts first came up with the idea in 1996, there was no other option but to build it himself!

If you or your friends have the handyman skills to piece together a treadmill desk on your own, you'll save money and have the satisfaction that comes with building something tangible.

But whether you choose to buy or to build, the real key is getting something that you'll use. That means making it accessible enough to work on every day and ergonomically comfortable enough that you can still accomplish what you need to for your work.

Popular Treadmill Desk Options

As the treadmill desk revolution picks up steam, more and more companies are entering the market. Here we'll explore several options at different price points so you can get an idea of what's available.

First, there are three summary spreadsheets to help give you a birds-eye view of the choices; one for desks only, one for treadmill bases only, and one for all-in-one treadmill desk set-ups.

The brands and products mentioned in this section are not an exhaustive list of every treadmill desk on the market, but rather are a representative sample of some popular options across the entire spectrum of price ranges. Prices shown are accurate at press time but are subject to change.

After that, the different brand selections are described in more detail.

Treadmill Work Desks (Desks Only)

Name	Price	Desktop Dimensions	Adjustable Height?
Tread-Top	$60	36" x 16"	No
TrekDesk	$479	72" x 34"	Yes
GeekDesk	$750	47" x 31"	Yes
NextDesk	$1,500	63" x 31"	Yes
TreadDesk	$1,530	36" x 28"	Yes

Treadmill Desk Bases (Treadmills Only)

Name	Price	Max. User Weight (lbs)	Max. Speed	Incline Mode?	Walking Surface	Warranty
LifeSpan	$816	300	4 mph	No	18" x 52"	3 years
TreadDesk	$955	320	4 mph	No	18" x 48"	2 years

All-in-One Treadmill Desks

Name	Price	Desktop Dimensions	Adjustable Height?	Max. User Weight (lbs)
Exerpeutic WorkFit	$728	48" x 24"	No	400
LifeSpan DT1200	$1,500	46" x 31"	Yes	350
SmartDesk Tower	$1,800	53" x 30"	Yes	250
TreadDesk All-in-One	$2,500	36" x 28"	Yes	320
Signature DZ9500	$2,200	63" x 32"	Yes	350
Steelcase Details Walkstation	$4,000	66" x 32"	Yes	350

Name	Max. Speed	Incline Mode?	Walking Surface	Warranty
Exerpeutic WorkFit	4 mph	Yes	20" x 40"	1 year
LifeSpan DT1200	4 mph	No	20" x 56"	3 years
SmartDesk Tower	4 mph	No	16" x 40"	1 year
TreadDesk All-in-One	4 mph	No	18" x 48"	2 years
Signature DZ9500	4 mph	No	20" x 56"	3 years
Steelcase Details Walkstation	2 mph	No	18" x 53"	3 years

Tread-Top

Tread-Top is a simple and portable desktop that rests on the handle bars of a treadmill. Initially, inventor Pamela Cawthorn found the lack of standardization in treadmills made it difficult to make a low-cost product that would work across a variety of models.

In fact, her treadmill desk experience pre-dates Dr. Levine and much of the "dangers of sitting" research. Beginning in 1999, Cawthorn experimented with a number of homemade variations for her home and office use, starting with a large tall table that stood over the treadmill.

Improving the design with each new version, she kept thinking to herself, "There's got to be a better way."

The answer came to her when she noticed a shift in treadmill design over the last decade. Nowadays, most treadmills feature fully horizontal handle bars that can accommodate a universal desktop, and with that, Tread-Top was born.

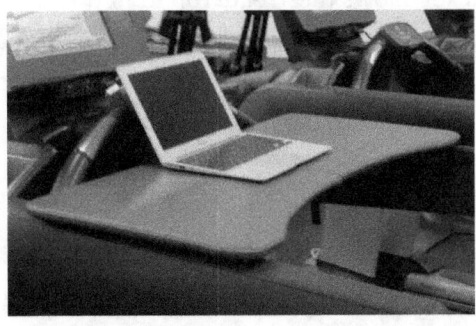

Tread-Top

The company began shipping Tread-Tops in 2012. The desktop is 3 feet wide by 16" deep, and attaches to the treadmill arms using Velcro straps. It weighs just 8 pounds and folds in half for easy storage and portability.

Currently, each desk is hand-made in Charlotte, North Carolina from pine shelving and coated with a durable customized decking treatment and finished with a light-grit spray-on epoxy.

The Tread-Top is available directly through their website (www.tread-top.com) and sells for $59.95 plus shipping. The low cost, ease of use, and portability are obvious advantages of the Tread-Top.

However, there are some drawbacks with the current model. For instance, it isn't compatible with older treadmill models that may not have perfectly horizontal handle arms. Also, the desktop surface is at a fixed height often resting much lower than other treadmill desk options, which may create comfort, usability, or ergonomics issues, especially for taller users.

Because the original intent for the Tread-Top was to be able to "fit any treadmill – new or old," Cawthorn addressed the issues above with the introduction of what she calls the "Universal Bracket."

The universal bracket allows the Tread-Top to fit on any treadmill by addressing the handle bar width and slope adjustment requirements. It's still not height adjustable, but does elevate the desktop roughly 6 inches, bringing it to a more comfortable height for taller walkers.

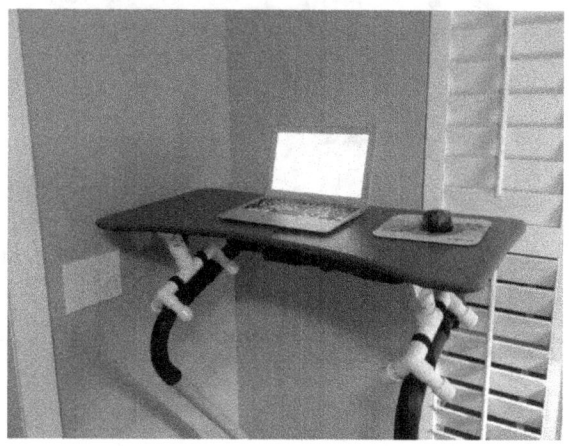

Tread-Top with universal bracket

The universal bracket is made of PVC pipe and Velcro, and creates a level surface to which the Tread-Top can be affixed to both parallel and sloped-armed treadmills. The any-angle PVC elbow allows the bracket to be adjusted to the slope of the treadmill arms. The universal bracket add-on costs about $30.

TrekDesk

TrekDesk was founded in 2008 and manufactures a U-shaped desk designed to stand over a treadmill. The desk itself is a massive 6 feet wide so the space required has to be a consideration. The height is adjustable to fit users between 5' 4" and 6' 4" and allow their hands to be at a comfortable working position.

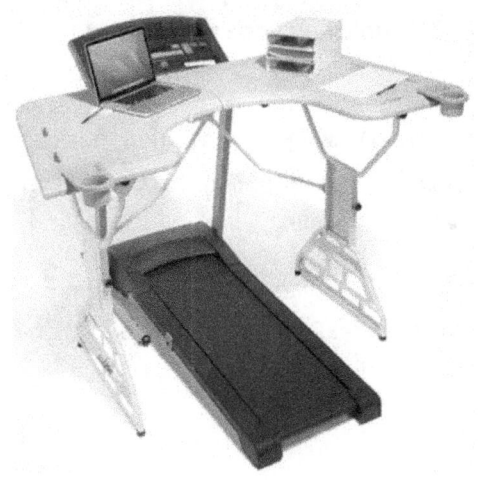

TrekDesk

The TrekDesk weighs in at just 57 pounds and can support nearly that much weight on its low-density polyethylene surface. Spread over its 6-foot wingspan, the plastic desktop and slender legs can feel cheap and flimsy. Several users have complained about a lack of stability and excessive vibration and wobbling.

One thing to consider with the TrekDesk is that it offers only one work surface so it may put a strain on your neck if forced to look down at the monitor the whole time. A workaround would be to mount an external LCD monitor on the wall behind the machine.

Because the desk is not fully integrated into the treadmill, and instead has to sit in front of the control panel, walkers will find themselves farther back on the belt. It's not a dealbreaker, but just something to be aware of, that could increase the small safety risk of falling off the back of the treadmill.

The benefit of being a standalone product is that you can use just about any treadmill as your base, maybe one you already have in your home or garage, or one you pick up on the cheap at a garage sale or on Craigslist.

The desk also includes 2 cup holders and a tri-level file organizer. Assembly is relatively simple and you can be up and walking in as little as 30-45 minutes.

All of this makes the TrekDesk a popular option. It is currently priced at $479 at Amazon (all prices mentioned in this book are subject to change without notice), with free shipping.

It should be noted that any similar adjustable-height desk could perform the same function as the TrekDesk so it might be worthwhile to shop around and see what else is out there.

Exerpeutic WorkFit

The Exerpeutic WorkFit line of treadmill desks is a mid-range option. The advantage over the TrekDesk is that it comes with a built-in treadmill, in case don't have access to one or don't want to be bothered with getting one separately.

The desk surface is 4 feet wide so it will accommodate a smaller footprint, and is collapsible for storage. Other thoughtful features include a desktop power outlet, padded wrist-rests, and speed controls on the extra-length handle bars.

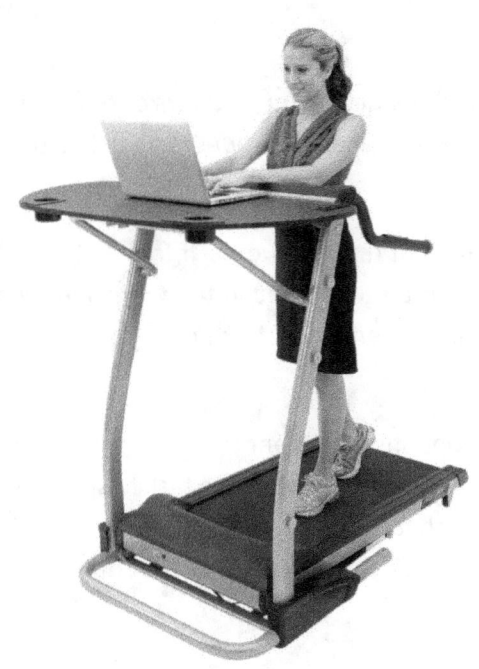

Exerpeutic WorkFit

The Exerpeutic WorkFit treadmill uses a quiet drive motor to limit noise pollution in your office, and adjusts up to a 15% incline. It maxes out at a top speed of 4 mph though, so it is designed purely for walking.

One drawback to the WorkFit station is that the desk height is fixed, meaning it might be too short for some walkers and too tall for others. And while the treadmill control panel is relatively compact, it does take up the prime real estate right at the front of the desk.

The treadmill belt itself is just 40 inches long, significantly shorter than the 52 to 55-inch standard found on other machines. This makes it a great choice to fit in a tight space but again can increase your risk of inadvertently falling off the back.

The WorkFit 2000 model is currently priced at $728 at Amazon. Despite its compact size, make sure you have someone to help you when it arrives; this treadmill desk weighs in at more than 160 pounds.

LifeSpan Fitness

LifeSpan is one of the leading manufacturers of treadmill desks. The brand was founded in 2002 and actually produces a full-line of exercise equipment.

One of the challenges of the do-it-yourself treadmill desk is figuring out what to do with the often-bulky and in-the-way control panel. LifeSpan addresses this issue but removing the upright portion of the treadmill entirely.

These standalone options are meant to be the perfect companion to a product like the TrekDesk, a tall standing task to span the front part of the treadmill. The detached control console comes with an 8' cord and will mount to whatever desk you choose to put over the top.

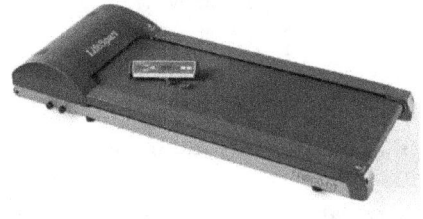

LifeSpan Treadmill Desk Base

These models range in price from around $800 - $2000 on Amazon and elsewhere. They are nice for their versatility, but on the high end the price is pretty steep to not even include the desk portion.

Thankfully, LifeSpan has you covered in that department as well if you're looking for an all-in-one alternative.

Their offerings include a sturdy desktop with robust metal legs. The desktop surface is a healthy 46 inches by 31 inches, and the height is adjustable to 16 different settings to accommodate walkers ranging from 4' 10" to 6' 8".

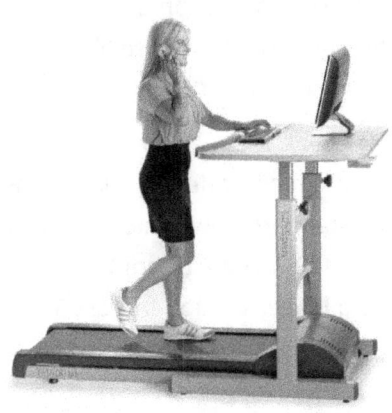

The Popular LifeSpan All-in-One Treadmill Desk

Because these workstations were specifically designed for office use, their motors are quieter than treadmills built for the gym. LifeSpan says that at 2 mph their treadmill should make less noise than your refrigerator!

Although the cup holders are missing on the current lineup, you'll still enjoy the padded armrests, super-compact control and display console, and thoughtful cable management tray in the back. The display keeps track of your speed, distance traveled, calories burned, and steps taken.

On the downside, the belt doesn't incline and the max speed is 4 mph so don't expect to be doing any running after work.

Still, the LifeSpan treadmill desks are among the most popular and award-winning models on the market. They typically range in price from around $1200 to $3000 depending on what features you're looking for. The top-of-the-line model comes with an electronically adjustable height mechanism with 2 memory pre-sets and Bluetooth integration so you can seamlessly track your exercise history online.

GeekDesk

GeekDesk sells a couple varieties of adjustable-height desks that are priced from around $750. They don't come with a treadmill but would be compatible with a standalone treadmill base like the LifeSpan model.

SmartDesk

SmartDesk offers two midrange treadmill desk options with electronic height adjustments. The standard Tower model costs around $1800 and comes with a 53" x 30" desktop and a treadmill base with a 47" belt. You can upgrade the base to a longer version for just $100, or to a more robust treadmill that can be used for both running and walking for just $200.

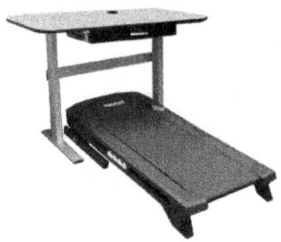

SmartDesk

With the SmartDesk, the treadmill controls are uniquely hidden in a desk drawer. The desktop is fully adjustable to accommodate a wide range of heights.

The other SmartDesk model, called the Shadow, is a longer rectangular shape to allow for a treadmill on one side and a chair on the other. Pricing starts around $2000.

TreadDesk

TreadDesk was founded in 2006 by Jerry Carr. After 20 years working in outside sales, Jerry suddenly found himself stuck in the office with a desk job. Immediately, he started putting on weight and feeling sluggish.

Carr knew he had to make a change and began experimenting with a treadmill in his office. Several protoypes later, TreadDesk was born.

Today, the company has several models to choose from, including a standalone treadmill similar to the LifeSpan model, adjustable height desks, and all-in-one packages.

Like the LifeSpan standalone treadmill, the TreadDesk base has a detached control panel and a maximum speed of 4 mph. These units are priced around $960 which includes shipping to the continental US. TreadDesk also includes a rubber floor mat free with each order that helps keep things clean and helps to dampen the treadmill noise.

The TreadDesk desks come in a variety of shapes and sizes ranging from 36" x 28" all the way up to 70" x 30". Should none of the existing models suit you, they have a custom-build option as well. The desktops are available in several different colors to match the existing décor of your office.

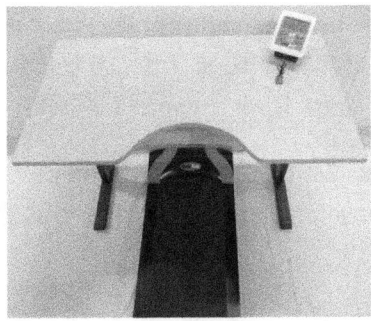

TreadDesk

The height of each desk is electronically adjustable with the push of a button. This is a major selling point because it means the same desk can potentially be used both for walking/standing, and for sitting. It also means it's great for use by teams of people with varying heights. Unfortunately this feature drives up the cost substantially; TreadDesk desks – *without the treadmill* – start around $1500.

The all-in-one packages merely combine the treadmill base with the desk of your choice, but there is a small price break for buying them together.

TreadDesk seems to be aiming more for the professional office environment rather than the home office user, though their products will certainly work equally well in both locations. Both the treadmill and desks are made in the USA. The belt and motor operate at a "whisper," just 35 decibels.

Pricing for the full treadmill and desk packages starts around $2500 and goes up to around $2800 for the largest desk. Shipping is free to the continental US and only a screwdriver is required for assembly.

NextDesk

NextDesk is a manufacturer of standing and adjustable-height desks based in Georgetown, Texas. Their desks are beautifully designed and they have several models that will fit over a treadmill base like the ones offered by LifeSpan.

While these desks are quite elegant, they don't come cheap, and the treadmill is sold separately (NextDesk offers a treadmill of their own that appears to be under license from LifeSpan for $999).

The Terra model comes with a 63" x 31.5" bamboo desktop and is available in 3 different colors. It is priced from $1497.

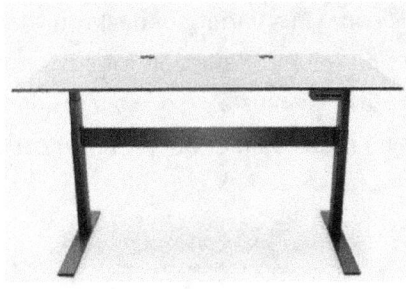

NextDesk

The NextDesk Air model takes a page out of Apple's playbook with its sleek metallic design and ultra-thin features. The surface is machined from a single piece of aluminum and is just ¼" thick. Pricing starts at $2178.

Each NextDesk is custom-manufactured on-demand in Texas based on your order date, so shipping times may vary depending on existing order volume. Customers can customize the colors, the keyboard platform, the cable management system, and the optional external monitor arm to really create a personalized product.

These power-adjustable desks change height at the push of a button using a quiet internal chain drive mechanism. If you're in a rush, the mechanism works smoothly at 1.7 inches per second.

An LED display shows the height and allows you to save three different presets into memory.

Still, without the treadmill, these are just standing desks. A complete package from NextDesk with a treadmill is around $2500 plus shipping.

Signature

The Signature DZ9500 claims to be the world's bestselling treadmill desk. It was once priced over $3000 but due to increased competition has been reduced to start at $2200 (plus shipping) at press time.

The Signature models come in a variety of desktop shapes, sizes, and colors, and they don't nickel-and-dime you for customizing your treadmill desk. The desktop surface is adjustable up to a maximum height of 54 inches, which should be more than enough to fit most users.

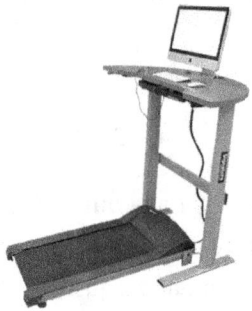

Signature

Signature offers the same three affordable treadmill base options as SmartDesk.

If you want to go all out with Signature though, they'll certainly let you. Their state-of-the-art flagship Craftsman desk is hand-crafted in Fort Wayne, Indiana, and this 75-inch beauty will set you back more than $5600. It features a fully adjustable-height luxurious desktop, a treadmill walking area, and a comfortable sitting area – for when you need a rest.

Steelcase Walkstation

At the top of the line is the Steelcase Details Walkstation. Steelcase has been in the office furniture business for over 100 years, and brings a wealth of experience into the Walkstation treadmill desk product.

This all-in-one offering includes a full-length commercial grade treadmill and an adjustable height desk – with the electronic height-adjustment mechanism integrated into the treadmill control panel.

The treadmill itself features a "whisper-quiet" motor built specifically for office environments. This is strictly a walking machine; the max speed is 2 mph and there is no incline option.

The desktop surface is available in two widths – 66" and 38" – and comes in several color options to match the existing look of your office. It includes a durable padded wrist-rest and sturdy steel legs to minimize vibration and wobbling. The removable display panel tracks your distance, calories burned, time, and speed.

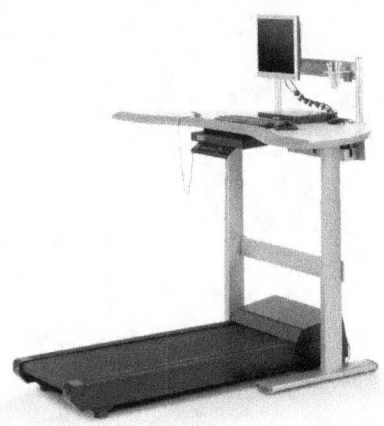

Steelcase Details Walkstation

The Walkstation is priced at roughly $4000, which includes a limited lifetime warranty from Steelcase (3 years on the treadmill parts). "White glove" shipping and installation charges of up to $300 may also apply, and may be helpful because the treadmill desk weighs over 200 pounds.The external monitor mounting arm and cable management system are available for an additional charge.

Steelcase also manufactures a combination walking-sitting workstation (not pictured) that includes an extra wide desktop. The treadmill will be on either the left or right side, and your chair on the other. With this set-up, you can easily stop the treadmill, adjust the height of the desk, and resume sitting when you need a break.

It eliminates the need to maintain 2 separate desks and has an efficient footprint if office space is a concern. The Sit-to-Stand model uses the same treadmill as the traditional Walkstation and has a suggested retail price of $4800.

Success Story #8: Walking Around the World

For 15 years, Jay Buster was a commodities trader on the floor of the Chicago Mercantile Exchange. The job was physically demanding and kept him on his feet all day long. On top of that, he walked to and from work, and didn't own a car.

Then Jay relocated to Boulder, Colorado and began a real estate development company. The work was challenging and rewarding, but he spent the majority of his time sitting at a desk. Despite regular exercise, the pounds slowly added on.

In 2007, Jay came across an article about Dr. Levine and his treadmill desk invention. By the end of the weekend, he had built one for himself.

The Desk

After learning about the treadmill desk, Jay immediately took to Craigslist to source an inexpensive treadmill. Next, he fashioned a makeshift desk (see the "Handle Bar Stack" method, described later) out of Styrofoam insulation and a thin sheet of melamine.

The Styrofoam was cut to rest across the handle bars of the treadmill, with several pieces stacked on top of each other. The material, which only cost about $20 from Home Depot, was lightweight and still sturdy enough to support the thin wooden or melamine topper, keyboard, and mouse. He attached dual monitors to the wall.

For the finishing touch, Jay painted the blue foam planks black with spray paint. "They were really ugly," he explains.

The Results

In the first four months of treadmill desk walking, Jay lost 16 pounds. Over the course of the next year, the total weight loss hovered around **20 pounds** as his body reached a healthy equilibrium.

He keeps one treadmill desk in his home office and another in his office at work. At home, his regular desk has been relegated to storage space. "I haven't used it in years; it's covered in dust," he adds.

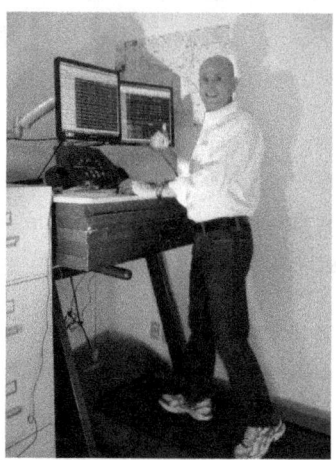

Jay's treadmill desk

The Miles

Jay racks up between 6 and 10 miles a day, 5 days a week, at a pace just over 1 mph.

Walking while working "takes some getting used to," he says. But after a while, the miles just start to go by. "It's shocking to see how far you can walk in a day, just doing your normal work."

By 2009, Jay had completed a 2500-mile virtual walk across the country from New York to Los Angeles. In another few years, he'll have gone far enough to fully circumnavigate the globe!

About Jay Buster

Jay Buster is a real estate investor based in Boulder, Colorado. In his spare time, he runs the popular website Treadmill-Desk.com, which is closing in on a million lifetime visitors.

On his site, he explains how to build an inexpensive treadmill desk of your own and shares other useful resources. But for Jay, the most rewarding aspect of maintaining the site is the thank you notes he receives from complete strangers, who credit his help with initiating amazing weight loss results and inspiring a healthier alternative to sitting all day.

DIY Treadmill Desk Tips and Strategies

Although there are some impressive Dr. Frankenstein creations on IkeaHackers and other DIY websites, building your own treadmill desk does not need to be a major project or require a master handyman to complete.

The basic elements are very simple: a treadmill and a desk.

In a perfect world, the treadmill will be a more modern, quieter model. And while we're in wish-list mode, it would great to have a detachable control panel or no upright portion at all. The tricky part in making a do-it-yourself treadmill is figuring out what to do with the bulky display panel that tends to get in the way of the desk.

The desk doesn't need to be anything fancy either. As we've seen, sometimes a simple platform to lay across the handle bars will do. A desk with an adjustable height would be best, but if the fixed height is perfect for you, and you're the only one using it, then it really doesn't matter.

With the desk, the most important thing is that it creates a stable surface to work on. There is no greater distraction than trying to focus on a wobbly computer screen.

For that reason, the best set up is to allow the treadmill and desk to both rest independently on the floor, rather than having the desktop attached to the treadmill. This arrangement offers the most stability and also the most flexibility when it comes time to move the treadmill desk.

Where to Shop for Parts?

For the treadmill desk builder, Craigslist is your best friend. You can find both used treadmills and desks in their "for sale" pages at bargain basement prices.

Garage sales, community rummage sales, and sites like Freecycle.org can also be great resources for finding low cost (or free) treadmills or desks.

For treadmills, you might consider stopping by the local gym to see if they have any equipment they're retiring.

What to Look For in a Used Treadmill?

In many cases, you'll find treadmills that are in almost new condition because of failed New Year's resolutions and other fitness plans that never really took hold.

But with treadmills, like any used electronics, it's best to do your homework before committing to a purchase. Your due diligence involves looking at the pictures the seller has provided, and searching for online reviews of the particular model being sold.

Even with treadmills that are several years old, you may still be able to find product reviews at Amazon or other online stores. Just search the model name and see what comes up. If a lot of people are complaining about technical problems or reliability issues, it might be wise to take a pass even if the price is attractive.

For professional reviews, check with Runner's World (www.runnersworld.com) or Treadmill Doctor (www.treadmilldoctor.com). Both sites have extensive and unbiased reviews of many different treadmill models.

Similarly, given the model of the treadmill, you can look up the cost of replacement parts online. The motor and the control panel will be the most expensive components and it's worth it to spend a few minutes checking out the parts cost in case your new treadmill decides to break on you a few weeks in.

The weight of the machine is a double-edged sword. The heavier models will offer more stability and may be better constructed, but will be more difficult to transport and move.

Consider your potential usage scenarios. Some treadmill desk treadmills max out at 2 mph, which is a perfectly good speed for working, but not so great if you want to use it for a jogging workout after hours. Along those same lines, some users swear by the incline feature for the added calorie-burning benefits, but not all treadmills offer incline capability.

When you go to check it out, plug it in and make sure it still works as described. Test it out yourself and play with the controls to verify their working condition. How loud is it?

And finally, it should be noted that most home-use treadmills aren't designed to hold up to being used for hours a day, even at low speeds. If you can find a commercial model or one specifically designed for treadmill desk-use, all the better.

What to Look for in a Desk?

When looking for desks, look for those with a height of at least 40 inches, and preferably adjustable even higher. Anything shorter than that and it may be very difficult to type, especially if you're on the taller side.

Also, consider the width footprint of the treadmill; the legs of the desk will need to be at least that far apart. Pay particular attention to the dimensions of the desktop surface – how will it fit in with the upright portion of the treadmill? If you have to make a cutout (see below), will you still have enough room to work?

There is no shortage of cheaply made office furniture out there, but here is one case where you'll definitely want something a little sturdier. That will mean heavier construction materials and more substantial supports and legs. Even though nobody is going to be sitting on top of the desk, you don't want to worry about its structural integrity.

Finding a suitable desk is a bit of a challenge, which explains why manufacturers can still command such price premiums for their treadmill desk offerings. But the aftermarket for these products is improving, as more and more standing desks and other treadmill desks are being sold each day.

Research the desks that will be a good fit for your treadmill and keep an eye on Craigslist. With a little patience, you'll find the perfect desktop.

What to Pay?

A decent used treadmill might run anywhere from $50 to $500 on Craigslist, so keep an eye out for one that fits your budget and sharpen up those negotiating skills.

You'll probably see a similar price range for desks, depending on the features and condition of the desk. Even though the desks have fewer moving parts, they seem to hold their value pretty well.

In most cases the old adage of "you get what you pay for" holds true, but there are always exceptions.

4 Popular Do-it-Yourself Treadmill Desk Models

Ready to get building? These common DIY treadmill desk models will get your creative juices flowing and you can see which one might deliver the best set-up for you.

The Imitation TrekDesk

Instead of paying $479 for the TrekDesk (shown earlier), you can opt to set up your own imitation version of it with any suitable standing desk. This is the simplest of all the do-it-yourself options and requires no special construction skills at all.

You simply need to find a standing desk that is stable, not too deep, and that you can position in front of the treadmill's control panel. The reason it can't be too deep is you still need to be able to reach the treadmill controls and don't want to be walking too far back on the belt.

The basic set-up is a tall, wide table that will straddle the arms of the treadmill and give you a nice surface to work on. If you're having a hard time finding a suitable tall desk, you may be able to fashion your own from inexpensive lumber or modify a regular desk to make it taller.

To extend the legs on a regular desk and still keep it sturdy, you could use 5-gallon buckets, milk crates, cinder blocks, or really any number of household items. With the imitation TrekDesk and these other DIY methods, the key is to experiment cheaply to find something that works well for your situation.

The Handle Bar Stack

The Handle Bar Stack is a variation on the Tread-Top we saw earlier, which laid a thin desktop platform across the handle bars of the treadmill. Since the height of the treadmill arm bars may be too low for many users to comfortably type, you can solve this issue by stacking lightweight foam insulation, wood, cardboard, books, or similar items on top of the base platform.

After you've achieved the desired height, just fasten a desktop to the top of the stack.

This method is obviously less-than-professional, but can get the job done in a home office set up. One potential pitfall here is if you elevate the desktop surface too high, it may be difficult to reach the controls behind it. Also, you may run into vibration issues by building directly on top of the treadmill arms.

Jay Buster of Treadmill-Desk.com (and Success Story #8) helped popularize The Handle Bar Stack by demonstrating his low-cost do-it-yourself job on his blog. The famous "$39 treadmill desk post" features pieces of 2" foam insulation paneling cut to the width of the treadmill handle bars (perhaps 40" wide by 12" deep) and stacked one on top of the other.

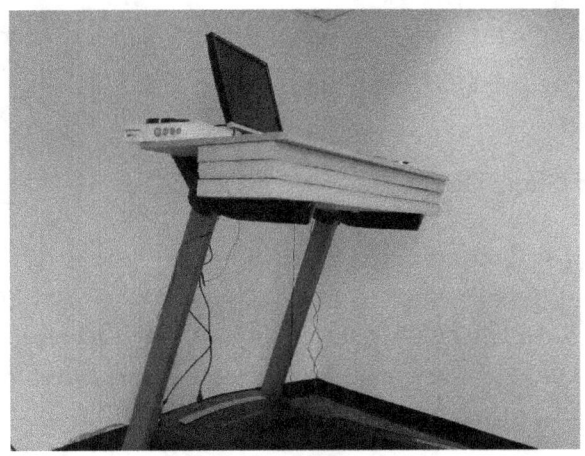

The famous $39 treadmill desk

Depending on your height and what constitutes a comfortable typing elevation for your hands, it could take 3-6 layers of the insulation. Luckily, a giant sheet of the stuff is only around $20 at Home Depot.

The desktop surface is a thin sheet of particleboard. It should also be available at the hardware store for less than $15. The drawback is it will probably need to be cut to size and fit around the control panel.

Jay recommends using a cardboard template to make your measurements on, and then using a jigsaw to cut along the pattern on the particleboard.

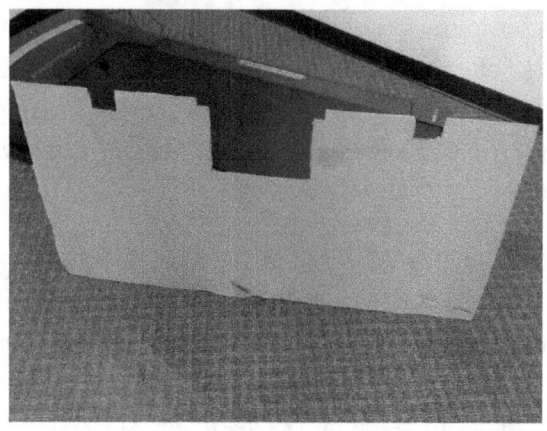

A sample cardboard treadmill desktop template

Once the wood is cut, simply lay it on top of the insulation stack. The particleboard is heavy enough that gravity alone is enough to keep it in place.

The Desktop Cutout Option

Sometimes, the choices of desks and treadmills leave you no option but to cut a hole in your desktop surface to accommodate the treadmill desk control panel. Placing the desk in front of the control panel would put you too far back on the belt and make it difficult to access the controls, and putting it over the top would make the desk too tall to use.

In this case, carefully measure out a hole in the desktop surface so that the desk could sit at the right height with the control panel sticking up through a portion. A popular desk model for this solution is the (discontinued) Ikea Jerker desk (look for it on Craigslist).

Cutting into the center of a piece of wood is more difficult than starting from an edge. You'll need to use a large drill bit to bore out a starter hole, which will give your handheld jigsaw a place to start cutting. If you want to get fancy, you can use a router to smooth out the edges.

It's best to first measure out the opening using a posterboard or cardboard template. That way you can make sure the dimensions are accurate before hacking up your desktop.

One thing to keep in mind if you're looking at the desk cutout option is the possibility the desk may have a lateral metal support bar on its underside. This would make it impossible to cut through for the purposes of fitting over the treadmill control panel.

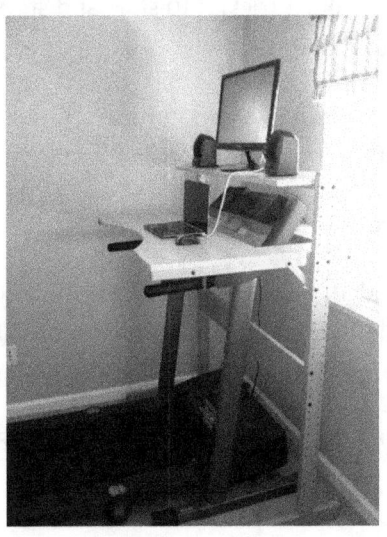

The author's desktop cutout treadmill desk

Check the IkeaHackers.net website for ideas and additional details.

The Wall Mount

With a little engineering, you can actually mount a flat panel monitor and desk surface to the wall. The advantages are you can position the monitor at an eye-level ergonomic height, and you won't have to worry about vibrations from the treadmill impacting either the desk surface or the monitor.

The brackets and supports for the desk should be able to support a lightweight piece of wood or plastic for the desktop, as well as the weight of your laptop and other working materials.

The problem is the upright portion of the treadmill still gets in the way. One creative solution is to flip the treadmill around, so the back of the belt is facing your wall-mounted desk surface and monitor, and reverse the polarity of the motor.

For most treadmill motors, this involves swapping the motor wires at the terminals on the circuit card. It's not rocket science but it's also not something I've personally done so I have a hard time recommending it to others. This also may make it trickier to start and stop, although I imagine you would get used to it over time.

The bigger downside with the wall-mounting set up is if you ever need to move your office, you're much more permanently "attached."

For Additional Inspiration

For additional low-budget treadmill desk ideas, just do a Google Image search (images.google.com) for "homemade treadmill desk." As you might imagine, you'll find an amazing assortment of ingenious contraptions.

And if nothing else, you'll get a good laugh at some of the more creative set-ups.

Success Story #9: Stepping and Pedaling to Weight Loss

As an accounting and tax advisor, Shannon Smit found herself trapped behind a desk most of the time. Aware of the health risks, she wore a pedometer and tried to walk the recommended 10,000 steps each day. But because of the work demands, meeting that activity level meant a 6am visit to the gym, which didn't always happen.

Shannon reasoned that the most elegant solution would be to somehow exercise while working. She took to Google and got the idea for a treadmill desk in early 2012.

The Desk

Shannon purchased a low cost treadmill for $189, which had the advantages of being lighter in weight and having a smaller frame, making it easier to fit under a desk.

She ordered a desk on eBay for $50; it was an adjustable Ikea model called the Frederik. While Ikea is still selling a desk under that name, the specific version popularly used for standing desks appears to be discontinued. (Why Ikea? Why?)

In addition to the treadmill workstation, Shannon also created a spin bike desk (see Treadmill Desk Alternatives) by positioning a stationary bike under the same Ikea desk. The only adjustment needed is to move the desktop to the next position higher to allow room for the bike handlebars.

The Results

Shannon was able to lose **28 pounds** over the course of a year.

"I walked an average of 1-2 hours per day, which is a lot more than I normally would," she explains. That small shift in work habit made a big impact on her health and her waistline.

The Speed

On the treadmill desk, Shannon keeps a pace of 1.5 mph. It's brisk enough to burn some calories but slow enough so that "you can still do work on the computer," she says.

On the bike, she'll average 9-10 mph, but explains, "It depends on the tension." (The spin bike has adjustable resistance to simulate climbing a hill.)

One advantage of the bike set up is it allows you to "work your body harder while still working," she adds. "Because it is a bike you can balance easier than the treadmill."

Are bike desks the next big thing?

The Shoes

"I just use some Asics."

About Shannon Smit

Shannon Smit is an accountant and tax advisor based in Melbourne, Australia. She founded Smart Business Solutions (www.smartbusinesssolutions.com.au) in 2006 after an accomplished career in the Big 4. When the company moves into a new office later this year, she'll be bringing the exercise desk with her so all the staff can take advantage of it.

Selling Your Boss on the Idea

For home office workers, you only need to convince yourself that a treadmill desk is a good idea. But for the rest of the world, there are likely going to be a few other decision-makers involved. As with any pitch, it's crucial to focus on the "what's in it for them" benefits.

Arm Yourself With Evidence

Because of the proliferation of news stories on the dangers of sitting, your boss may already be well aware of the risks of a sedentary lifestyle. Still, a summary of the available data will only strengthen your case. Feel free to use the data cited in the beginning of this book to help make your appeal. (There is also a list of sources at the very end.)

Don't Go At It Alone

Safety in numbers, right? It makes sense to gather a consensus among your co-workers and make sure they are on board with the treadmill desk request. If management understands that a large number of employees are asking for the change, they should be more likely to comply.

You may ask co-workers to sign a "walking pledge", start a treadmill desk petition, or even initiate an office-wide "Biggest Loser" contest like we saw at Charles River Apparel.

An Investment, Rather Than a Cost

Asking your boss to install potentially several thousand dollars worth of new office furniture is understandably a tough sell. That is why it is important to promote the treadmill desk (or desks) as an investment – not a cost, even though the tangible returns may not be monetary.

And the truth is a treadmill desk *is* an investment. It's an investment in the health of the company's employees; in their well-being, happiness, and productivity.

Happier employees tend to turnover less frequently and companies with strong employee retention benefit from significantly lower recruitment and training costs.

In the long run, the company may also realize reduced health insurance costs as the benefits of a healthier workforce takes hold.

Worker's Compensation Risk

California-based ergonomics consultant Vanessa Friedman says employers are more apt to consider the treadmill desk investment after they're faced with a costly worker's compensation claim. For example, if an employee claims their sedentary work environment caused their back injury, the settlement might cost $60,000 if the workplace is found liable. "After that, $1,500 on a desk doesn't seem like a lot to spend," Friedman explains.

And while the veiled threat of litigation isn't usually the best route to get what you want, it is a possible outcome that employers should be aware of. It sounds crazy, but it happens. Installing a treadmill desk or two might be enough to show they are making an effort to provide a healthy and ergonomic workplace.

Start Small

Instead of asking to replace an entire floor of cubicles, propose a more palatable investment of one or two treadmill workstations. Also, take care to note they will be made available for everyone to use on a shared basis, not just dedicated to assigned employees.

If the idea is seen as a low-risk trial, rather than a full-scale office overhaul, it is far more likely to gain acceptance. After a couple months, if demand for treadmill time is strong, you can broach the subject of adding more.

Did You Know?

In Denmark, employers are legally required to provide adjustable desks for their staff.

Treadmill Desk Alternatives

Not quite ready to commit to the full treadmill desk experience? Thankfully there are a few alternatives that are still an improvement over sitting the entire day.

Standing Desks

The concept of a standing desk has been around for centuries. In fact, some of history's most prolific figures were known to use standing desks, including Leonardo da Vinci, Thomas Jefferson, and Winston Churchill.

Although standing will not burn nearly as many calories as walking, it still engages your leg muscles and is healthier than sitting. As mentioned in the previous sections, a number of standing desk options are available at varying costs and qualities.

Sit-Stand Desks

To be fair, standing all day may not be realistic. It can get tiring and uncomfortable, even for the most physically fit individuals. One solution is the sit-stand desk, an adjustable height desk that lets you alternate between sitting and standing at your convenience.

Most of the sit-stand desks on the market include an electronic adjustment mechanism to easily change the height. However, this additional technology increases their cost. A number of the desks explored earlier could be used as sit-stand desks by simply leaving out the treadmill.

Exercise Ball Chairs

A growing trend is to replace traditional office chairs with large inflatable exercise balls. The theory is by sitting on these balls, workers will have to engage their core stabilizing muscles more.

However, studies have shown the practical impact of exercise ball chairs to be negligible. In fact, workers only burn an extra 4 calories an hour over traditional office chairs – not enough to trigger any serious body changes.

That said, sitting on a relatively unstable surface such as an exercise ball can help stimulate brain function and keep employees more alert, so all is not completely lost.

Bike Desks

Similar to a treadmill desk, a bike desk (like the one employed by Shannon in Success Story #9) simply replaces the treadmill with an exercise bike or other pedal mechanism beneath the desk surface. Bike desks have the advantage of keeping your legs moving and muscles working throughout the day, while still being able to maintain a potentially more comfortable seated position.

The most popular all-in-one bike desk model is made by FitDesk, shown in the picture below. It is currently priced around $250 at Amazon.com, making it much more affordable than even some of the lower-end treadmill desks.

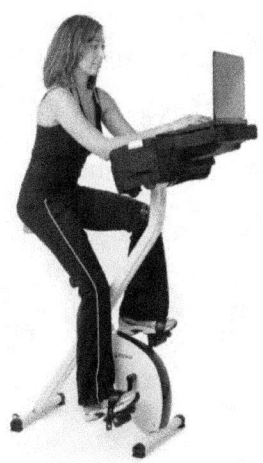

FitDesk Bike Desk

Success Story #10: The 100 Pound Club

Mutual of Omaha was one of the first major companies to install treadmill desks in their office, back in 2008. They wanted to study firsthand the impact the walking workstations would have on employee's health and productivity.

As an insurance provider, it made perfect sense to take the lead in a sweeping workplace health trend.

The Desks

Mutual of Omaha's treadmill desk experiment began with 4 Steelcase Walkstations, which cost around $4000 each.

The Results

Almost immediately, employees who used the treadmill desks began to report lower cholesterol, lower blood pressure, and improved productivity.

Call center manager Brandi Hanson has lost an incredible **130 pounds** by incorporating the treadmill into her daily work schedule. Before she started walking, Hanson exhibited common symptoms of "sitting disease." She was overweight, felt sluggish, and lacked energy.

To drop all that weight without making any other drastic lifestyle changes, "It just makes me feel amazing," Hanson said.

The Miles

Hanson puts in 8 miles a day on her treadmill desk, and together Mutual of Omaha employees have racked up tens of thousands of miles since 2008.

About Mutual of Omaha

Mutual of Omaha is a Fortune 500 provider of insurance and financial services. The Omaha, Nebraska company was founded in 1909 and is considered a leader in workplace health initiatives, in part due to their early adoption of treadmill desks.

A Growing Community

There is an online social network for treadmill desk walkers called Office Walkers (officewalkers.ning.com). The group began in 2008 and is now over 1000 members strong!

You'll find helpful forum discussions, treadmill reviews, DIY support, and a friendly community of current and future treadmill desk jockeys.

Conclusions

We're just at the beginning of the treadmill desk revolution. Momentum is gaining as more and more people become aware of the long-term dangers of their sedentary work habits.

Sitting is lethal. But there is an alternative, and it doesn't have to break the bank – though you can certainly spend the money if you have it.

Thousands of people have made the switch, taking those first proactive steps to stop "sitting disease." Those who've shared their stories here are only the tip of the iceberg.

We've seen how walking while you work is a small change that creates a ripple effect through your whole life. It creates a positive energy and a healthier outlook both in and out of the office.

There's no doubt: our work will still involve computers for the foreseeable future. But if we change how we interface with those computers we can build a healthier nation and planet.

About the Author

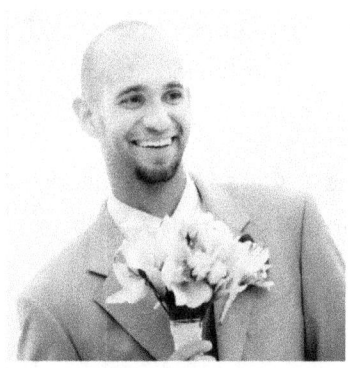

Nick Loper is an online entrepreneur and lifelong student in the game of business. He lives in Northern California with his wife Bryn and a lovable giant Shih-Tzu called Mochi. On a typical day you can find him writing, working on his latest business idea, rooting for the Mariners, or skiing the Sierra pow.

This book was written over the course of 68.7 miles on Nick's home office treadmill desk, which he installed in 2011.

The treadmill and desk were both sourced on Craigslist for about $120 each. The only other expense was $20 for a fifth of Jack Daniels and a roll of masking tape to repay a friend for letting him borrow the necessary tools and lending his handyman expertise. (To be fair, Bryn the engineering wife helped with the design as well – and took the cover photo for this book.)

Nick logs at least 30 miles a week and has had several "double-digit-days" of 10 miles or more. He started out at 1 mph, and gradually increased it over the course of the first year to 2 mph.

He alternates between 3 choices of shoes: a pair of Salomon trail runners, a pair of Chaco sandals, and (somewhat embarrassingly) a pair of Crocs canvas shoes.

Want to know more? Drop by and say hi at his personal blog (sidehustlenation.com), or follow him on twitter (twitter.com/nloper).

Do you have a treadmill desk success story to share? Get in touch and you might just be featured in a future version of this book!

Also by Nick

Nick is also the author of:

Virtual Assistant Assistant: The Ultimate Guide to Finding, Hiring, and Working with Virtual Assistants

Thank You

I'd like to say a quick "thank you" for purchasing this book.

Obviously there are thousands of books about health and weight loss, but you took a chance and chose this one.

Hopefully it got the gears turning with a unique approach to work and weight loss, and you got some inspiration from the success stories included.

So thank you for downloading the book and reading all the way to the end.

If you liked what you read, I need your help!

Please take a minute to leave a quick review on Amazon.

The feedback is really valuable because it will guide future editions of this book and I'm always striving to improve my writing. Thanks for your help!

Treadmill Desk Resources

This section is a compilation of the websites mentioned in the book, plus a few extras that are worth checking out.

ApartmentTherapy.com – A popular site with a number of treadmill desk posts over the years.

Craigslist.org – The go-to source for used treadmills and a great place to look for desks too.

FitBit.com – A sleek pedometer with a beautiful online interface to help track your steps and your weight loss goals.

IkeaHackers.net – Great resource for transforming Ikea furniture into standing desks and treadmill desks.

ModTable – A series of adjustable height desks starting around $550.

Officewalkers.ning.com – A social network (or support group!) for treadmill desk walkers.

RunnersWorld.com – Unbiased treadmill reviews.

Tread-Top.com – Inexpensive desktop that affixes the handle bars of any treadmill.

Treadmill-Desk.com – Jay Buster's treadmill desk blog. Home of the $39 treadmill desk.

TreadmillDeskDiary.com – A well-written personal blog with weight loss charts, detailed pictures, tips, and more.

TreadmillDoctor.com – Unbiased treadmill reviews, replacement parts, and repair help.

VersaDesk.com – Adjustable height desks that rest on top of your current desk, starting at just $275.

WorkWhileWalking.com – A treadmill desk blog with useful articles and reviews of popular treadmill desk models.

Sources

All product images courtesy of their respective sellers.

American Time Use Survey. Bureau of Labor Statistics, November 2012.

Americans Spend 34 Hours a Week Watching TV. New York Daily News, September 2012.

Britons Spend More Than 14 Hours a Day Sitting Down. The Telegraph, May 2010.

Can You Move it and Work it on a Treadmill Desk? NPR, November 2012.

Employees Workout While They Work at Omaha Company. KETV, February 2012.

Future Workplaces Will Function Best with Stone Age Features, UC Berkeley Professors Suggest. University of California Berkeley, August 2000.

Get Up. Get Out. Don't Sit. New York Times, October 2012.

The Good and Bad of Walking While Working. Popular Mechanics, October 2012.

Historical Timeline: Farmers and the Land. AG Classroom.

How I Keep My Job From Killing Me. Inc., August 2012.

I Put In 5 Miles at the Office. New York Times, September 2008.

I Tried It: Treadmill Desk. Philadelphia Magazine, September 2012.

Kill Your Desk Chair and Start Standing. BusinessWeek, June 2012.

The New Key to Office Productivity? Walking. Greatist, January 2013.

Paul Salopek: Going For a Seven-Year Walk. BBC, January 2013.

Sitting Less May Be Key for Maximum Longevity. Mercola, November 2012.

Study: Multi-business Study of the Effect of Low Impact Physical Activity on Employee Health and Wellbeing. Lancaster University, 2011

Treadmill Desks: How Practical Are They? BBC, January 2013.

Treadmill Desks May Help Get Office Workers Moving. Las Vegas Review-Journal, October 2011.

Treadmill Desks Might Be the Next Office Health Trend. Yahoo News, November 2012.

Walking While You Work. Forbes, April 2013.

Why Sitting at Work Can Be So Deadly. Forbes, May 2012.

Why Sitting Increases Your Risk of Dying Sooner. Forbes, February 2013.

Your Treadmill Desk is Hurting Your Productivity. Business Insider, January 2013.

That's all folks. Time to get walking!

www.ingramcontent.com/pod-product-compliance
Lightning Source LLC
Chambersburg PA
CBHW070556290526
45790CB00002B/717